STRESS MANAGEMENT
How to cope up with stress and brings joy in life naturally

What is Stress?

Stress is response of our body to any kind of change related to events and actions that are going on around us. Our body could respond physically, mentally or emotionally.

When we are stressed, our body releases variety of chemicals into our blood in order to prepare us for physical action. As a result, at the moment of danger, blood can change its course from unnecessary functions of body. Thus, we may have more energy and strength that could help us in case of physical threat.

As stated above, stress could be related to our emotions. The response of our body to both physical and emotional anxiety is the same. In other words, blood flow is restricted to those parts of our body, that has unnecessary functions to overcome stress. Hence, if the stress is caused by emotional events, the functionality of our brain is reduced. As a consequence, we may be limited to think conservatively.

What Causes Stress?

There is no universal cause of stress. We all have different psychological state, and we perceive situations differently. Thus, the situation that may cause one person to be stressed, does not necessarily will have the same effect on other person. However, situations or events that cause stress have common feature. When people have the sense of inability to manage pressure that is put on them, they feel stressed.

THE ROOTS OF STRESS

1. LESS LEISURE TIME

Many people often associate stress with having to deal with childcare and taking care of the household.

However, if we were to compare the amount of time that people spend taking care of their homes and families now with the amount of time spent doing the same things back in the 1910's, we would arrive at the same average number of hours per week: 52 hours.

The reason for this is that we are now spending more time on additional activities such as grocery shopping and people don't usually find these activities as leisurely.

So even if we have plenty of modern appliances to lessen the time needed to complete different tasks, the time that we could spend for leisure is now being consumed by additional, unavoidable activities and chores.

2. STRESSORS ABOUND

In an ideal world, a person who continually feels stressed at work would be able to unwind and distress when he comes home.

I'm sure there are some people who have managed to accomplish this feat and I am also certain that they are extremely happy that they "cracked the code".

However, for 60% of adult Americans, the scenario isn't as bright and stress free. The present reality is that more than 50% of all adults in America experience the same level of stress both at home and at work. That means that an ordinary working adult no longer experiences a reprieve from stress because both environments are deemed stressful.

3. HARMFUL SOCIETAL STANDARDS

It is no secret that modern society is still ruled by double standards, especially in the workplace.

Despites significant breakthroughs in the field of gender equality, many people still subscribe to the idea that a woman who is too independent and forward-thinking is undesirable.

On the flipside, a man who doesn't show the same set of skills is also considered a failure in terms of his professional character.

These double standards are actually toxic in the workplace because it encourages aggressive competition in males but fails to reward females who show drive and initiative. This can make the workplace an extremely frustrating and stressful place for both males and females.

4. CHRONIC OVERWORK

More than 25% of all adult working Americans complain of not having enough time in a day to finish everything they have to do.

To compensate for the scarcity of time, many adults resort to overworking which usually leads to a "burn out" phase. It can be difficult to recover from burn out if nothing is actively done to reduce a person's stress levels at home and at work.

5. FRAGMENTATION

The present divorce rate in the United States is a staggering 50%. This means that a significant percentage of the entire American population is comprised of single-parent families with only 1 main earner.

This reality is forcing many single parents (mostly females) to work twice or thrice as hard just to keep up with the daily expenses of their families.

Obviously this situation is extremely stressful because leisure time is almost nonexistent and all other free time from work is diverted to taking care of the children and household.

Acknowledgement

I am writing this book about how to deal with stress efficiently and naturally.
Stress occurs when you perceive that demands placed on you — such as work, school or relationships — exceed your ability to cope. Some stress can be beneficial at times, producing a boost that provides the drive and energy to help people get through situations like exams or work deadlines. However, an extreme amount of stress can have health consequences, affecting the immune, cardiovascular and neuroendocrine and central nervous systems, and take a severe emotional toll.

Untreated chronic stress can result in serious health conditions including anxiety, insomnia, muscle pain, high blood pressure and a weakened immune system. Research shows that stress can contribute to the development of major illnesses, such as heart disease, depression and obesity.

But by finding positive, healthy ways to manage stress as it occurs, many of these negative health consequences can be reduced. Everyone is different, and so are the ways they choose to manage their stress. Some people prefer pursuing hobbies such as gardening, playing music and creating art, while others find relief in more solitary activities: meditation, yoga and walking.

Here are five healthy techniques that psychological research has shown to help reduce stress in the short- and long-term.

Take a break from the stressor. It may seem difficult to get away from a big work project, a crying baby or a growing credit card bill. But when you give yourself permission to step away from it, you let yourself have time to do something else, which can help you have a new perspective or practice techniques to feel less overwhelmed. It's important to not avoid your stress (those bills have to be paid sometime), but even just 20-minutes to take care of yourself is helpful.

Exercise. The research keeps growing — exercise benefits your mind just as well as your body. We keep hearing about the long-term benefits of a regular exercise routine. But even a 20-minute walk, run, swim or dance session in the midst of a stressful time can give an immediate effect that can last for several hours.

Smile and laugh. Our brains are interconnected with our emotions and facial expressions. When people are stressed, they often hold a lot of the stress in their face. So laughs or smiles can help relieve some of that tension and improve the situation.

Get social support. Call a friend, send an email. When you share your concerns or feelings with another person, it does help relieve stress. But it's important that the person whom you talk to is someone whom you trust and whom you feel can understand and validate you. If your family is a stressor, for example, it may not alleviate your stress if you share your works woes with one of them.

Meditate. Meditation and mindful prayer help the mind and body to relax and focus. Mindfulness can help people see new perspectives, develop self-compassion and forgiveness. When practicing a form of mindfulness, people can release emotions that may have been causing the body physical stress. Much like exercise, research has shown that even meditating briefly can reap immediate benefits

Forgive: Do Forgiveness Practice

Forgiveness is a choice not something that you learn over time. It starts with understanding that God has forgiven us through Jesus Christ our Saviour and He says that unless we forgive others their sins we can not receive His forgiveness. That's because forgiveness is a channel that flows both ways so you can't have it flowing in without it flowing out. It has nothing to do with you deeming a person worthy - in many cases this will never be the case. Likewise we would not have been deemed worthy of God's forgiveness, it is simply a gift and so we must give it to others as a gift. This is so that we can be free to move forward.

Forgiveness begins with willing to do so and thus with the mouth……..you need to begin by confessing that forgiveness verbally out loud. As Paul said in the book of Romans, "call those things that be not as though they were". Forgiveness will never be something you feel initially. You speak out loud that you forgive [name] for [action]. [At this point it is very important to ignore any anxiety, and in some cases rage, that comes with the words.]

Speak out loud the name of the person and say,

I am sorry.
Please forgive me.
Thank you.
I love you.

Practice it daily 15 minutes in the morning and 10 minutes in the night. You will feel much better. Speaking the name and action are very important. What you speak goes into your spirit where the seed takes root and with continual watering (repeat process) begins to grow. Most important when we commit to forgive, God empowers our actions to help us. At some point the negative energy from the experience will be released from your spirit and soul and then you will know that the forgiveness has been completed. It will be felt in your spirit and in many cases the release from the soul is manifest in your physical well being. (Unforgiveness shows up in the body like putting on a garment.) And then the burden is gone and it simply becomes a memory with no current connection. That is why forgiveness is so freeing.

Disclaimer: This book is not intended as a substitute for the medical advice of physicians. The reader should regularly consult a physician in matters relating to his/her health and particularly with respect to any symptoms that may require diagnosis or medical attention.

Chapter- 1

The power of forgiveness

Acceptance.

Acceptance is the core power by which one can forgive completely. Complete forgiveness whether for your friend, your ex, your family member, or even for yourself, is essential to get rid of the mental anguish and emotional burden that one may carry if they don't learn how to forgive.

For that to happen, you must first accept the reality as it is and not deny it, accept that we don't need to attach expectations to everyone or everything in life.

Accept the fact that every action of yours or others' doesn't always need a 'Should have' or a 'What if'.

Accept that mistakes of others' or even yourself are necessary to guide you in life and make you a better person with more lessons, and then you'll learn to forgive and realize that you aren't running away from accepting the reality, and you are brave enough to forgive in a world wherein people are weak enough to take revenge or hold on to emotions/things/people just because they didn't forgive or accept.

There's a quote; "Only the Brave and the Broken know how to forgive."

"If you forgive men when they sin against you, your heavenly Father will also forgive you. But if you do not forgive men their sins, your Father will not forgive your sins."

"The truth is, unless you let go, unless your forgive yourself, unless you forgive the situation, unless you realize that the situation is over, you cannot move forward."

"Hurt people hurt people. That's how pain patterns get passed on, generation after generation. Break the chain today. Meet anger with sympathy, contempt with compassion, cruelty with kindness. Greet grimaces with smiles. Forgive and forget about finding fault. Love is the weapon of the future."

"Don't forget what you camc out of, but keep your eye's on the Lord! Our resentments will keep us sick; they are the number 1 offender. Forgiveness is powerful for the person forgiving - Set that bag of bricks down before God and let Him take that burden from you; and He will give you Peace."

Ho'oponopono is a wonderful forgiveness method with

deep roots in the beautiful spirit of the Hawaiian culture. The Four Steps to Forgiveness is a new secular method and has no particular cultural or religious associations. People use it as-is or they modify it to fit their religious or culture needs. Four simple phrases are:

I am sorry.
Please forgive me.
Thank you.
I love you.

Practice it daily in the morning for 10 minutes and 10 minutes in the night before going to bed. It works wonder.

Ho'oponopono is an ancient Hawaiian practice for forgiveness and reconciliation. It's more than the prayer alone; it's a process of making things right in your relationships -- with others, ancestors, deities, the earth, yourself.

The family ritual focuses on working through problems together, openly expressing feelings, and releasing each other. It's the act and intention of holding a space for reflection, repentance, forgiveness, and gratitude.

Special words are exchanged, emotions are revealed, and forgiveness flows both ways. A ceremonial feast might follow, symbolizing the release.

The philosophy behind this practice is that we're each responsible for what shows up in our reality. We own our feelings and our experiences. So even if someone else has wronged us, we're the ones saying "I am sorry. Forgive me..."

The foundation of this practice is unity: an unbreakable bond connects you to everyone else, even though we seem so separate.

When errors are corrected externally, errors are corrected internally. When you "cleanse" your consciousness, you contribute to the cleansing of the "collective consciousness." When you forgive others, you, too, are forgiven.

Loving each other and loving yourself is kind of the same thing.

When you focus on healing the past, you help heal your life right here, right now. When you right any wrongs in your thinking, you adjust and amend problems in the physical realm.

The practice of Ho'oponopono helps you understand and heal the experiences in your life that you've "attracted" or participated in, or have been affected by.

There are four forces at work in this prayer: repentance, forgiveness, gratitude, and love. These are reflected in the four phrases that make up the prayer.

The phrases, which you can repeat in any order, silently to yourself or out loud, are:

I am sorry.
Please Forgive me.
Thank you.
I love you.
It's natural to resist this practice at first, especially if you've got a lot of healing to do. After a few times, it gets easier.

You might feel better right away, or feel your evolution like a slow melt into love.
All of us not only have healing powers within us, but we activate and use them much of the time. We must remember that our body and mind are constantly in a a healing with themselves. We would never have made it through childhood if they were not. The biggest challenge is realizing that we are the ones who are doing most of the healing and are only assisted by outside people and modalities.

Unfortunately, we tend to think or believe that it is the person or thing outside of us that is doing the bulk of the healing. Nothing could be further from the truth. No doctor, surgery, medicine or therapy (holistic or conventional) could possibly do all of it; rather, it is our own internal energy that is utilizing these outside influences to their fullest degree to achieve a recovery. I believe that this must be true because not all patients will fully recover or even survive, although the outer influences believe that they should.

The core of the matter lies in our participation with the ailment or disease and our internal belief in the outer person or thing that has come to heal us. The physical outer manifestations are giving us inner healing support. Which way the tide may turn depends upon the individual's relationship to themselves, the chosen treatments and modalities and to the disease itself. If this combination bodes well, the outcome may be favorable.

Unfortunately, because many of us have been previously programmed to believe or not believe that certain practices or institutions are correct versus others, we force ourselves into a prison of beliefs that may or may not be of benefit to us. Our minds become tricked into following what we SHOULD do even though it goes against our internal desire of what we would LIKE to do. This can be detrimental to the outcome of the situation and may end in with undesirable consequences.

Chapter-2

Limiting beliefs are the biggest culprit of stress

What are limiting beliefs?
Limiting beliefs are those which limit us in certain ways
to do the things. Due to our limiting beliefs only if
started to think I am not good enough. I can't do that. It
is not meant for me.

Limiting beliefs are often about our selves and our self-identity. The beliefs may also be about other people and the world in general.

In any case, they set the boundaries for us.

First you need to identify your limiting beliefs. Many people will tell you that this is difficult. It isn't.

You just need to figure out where in your life you're limiting yourself needlessly:

Where do you want to do something but don't, for whatever reason?
Where do you want to not do something, but do, for whatever reason?
When you hit some kind of limit, there's often a belief which defines that limit.

Secondly, you need to tease out the entire limiting belief.

This is also easier than you might think and doesn't require a lot of introspection, or soul-searching.

Beliefs have the form: If X then Y which means Z

For example, "If I try, then I'll fail, which means I'm a failure"

So go back to the things you identified in the first part.

If you did do the thing you don't normally do, what would happen?
This gives you the 'if X then Y' part.

Next, ask yourself what it would mean if that happened. That will give you the 'which means Z' part.

Finally, you need to 'challenge' the limiting belief, or have someone else do that for you.

Fortunately, there are some general patterns which help to create change in a limiting belief. Here are two of them:

(i) Counter-example

Limiting beliefs are built from examples. If you can offer valid examples which don't lead to the limiting belief, you can begin to open up their world.

You'll need a number of good counter-examples, because one exception 'proves the rule'. Several exceptions show the belief is really shaky and requires redefinition.

(ii) Exaggerate

Sometimes a really vivid counter-example can make all the difference, so feel free to exaggerate to make your case:

"All dogs are scary? Even Scooby Doo?"

If you can get someone to laugh about their problems, you're already most of the way to changing them.

NOTE: When you challenge another person's limiting belief, be as gentle as you can. We're talking about the underpinnings of their reality here.

To summarise:

Limiting beliefs can be easy to identify and define fully.

Once you have done that, you can often see what you need to do to break them down - the cracks will begin to show.

Then you can overturn them and redefine your limits in the process.

We all believe our New Year's resolutions, and Vows to each other. It's the inability to keep them operative that lets us down.

The mass-culture pundits all pretend that merely introducing people to concepts will be sufficient to overcome psychological, or belief, limitations. The largely unschooled mass audience believes them, and wonder why their lives return to usual after one to three months.

Once I recognized that I was hurting my life with my own decisions, I started to look around into both paid, and unpaid, sources of that kind of help. The paid stuff was powerful, and gave me an optimism buzz, that then wore off. The unpaid stuff was almost as good. Everyone's life is about the book they are reading at the moment. That's what happens because the next occasion for doubt, or anger, or jealousy, or fear, or brain dumps, are just around the corner. Then life returns to the before temp-buzz paths.
This sounds ludicrous, yet is bitter, and destroys lives.
A life is just as destroyed when repeated disappointment in failed efforts to improve result in resignation, and all of its ugly scenarios.

That reality was the motivation for many brilliant people in India, China, Japan, to come up with a way for people to reliably, in a self-directed fashion, without shaving their heads, or going to live in some colony, dissolve the limiting, and destructive beliefs.

There was progress, and that resulted in the founding of a group, in 1930, whose sole goal is world peace, and prosperity, through individual happiness. Here's a description of the method, and some concepts that underlie it.

Average persons often have far more ability to produce great results than they know.

The things that stop most people from being great are emotional, rather than cognitive blockages. If you can get skilled therapy, great, then the blocks can be dealt with in a systematic, and reliable way, by combining the therapy with this information.

If you can't get skilled therapy for your emotional blocks, you can still progress. Just get help from a senior practitioner who has used the method outlined below.

Here's some cognitive help.

1. You are unique, and so is everyone else.

Keeping this in mind will protect you from cultural, ethnic prejudice.

2. You need more than just yourself, in order to live, and so does everyone else.

Keeping this in mind will protect you from spoiling your relationships, and environment.

3. There are things you know, and a wholc lot you don't. That's true for everybody.

Keeping this in mind protects you from feeling inadequate.

4. Nothing happens, unless the conditions for it to happen are right.

This knowledge help to understand origins.

5. What goes around, comes around.

This simple sentence keeps you from making false assumptions about what to do.

6. Lives change, yet LIFE goes on.

This very powerful bit wisdom help to reduce the pain of impermanence.

7. We Don't Have to Be Perfect in Whatever We Do
This might sound obvious, but, I was raised by strict, middle-class Indian parents who only had only one dream for me — that I should have a future better than their present. To make this dream become a reality, they had sky-high expectations from me in whatever endeavour I attempted. Be it art competitions, dance classes, martial arts training, or school exams; I had to ace them all. If I didn't, they would make it clear how disappointed they were in me and how I had failed them.
These expectations continued to haunt me in my adult life, leading me to believe that no matter what I attempt in life, I had to succeed.
Don't get me wrong. Being ambitious is not bad.
But, wanting to win at everything to the extent that you fill yourself with guilt and brutal self-retribution each time you fail is toxic not just to your mental health, but to your emotional and physical health as well.
Failure in a small project that won't even matter in the ultimate scheme of things can bring your confidence down and make you feel like you aren't good enough. That just because you failed in one project, you are a failure.
The truth is — you are not.
Every individual has their own strengths and weaknesses, and in the limited time that you have on earth, the best you can do is play to your strengths.

The endeavours that don't bring tangible results — let them go. Work on the ones that you are good at and keep improving till there's no one better at it than you. After all, no one wants to end up like the old proverb — "Jack of all trades, master of none."

8.Making Mistakes Doesn't Make Us A Bad Person
You are only human. You can stop blaming yourself for that time you fucked up. Yes, I know you ended up hurting yourself and other people, but that was not in your hands. You did the best you could in the situation you were in. You don't have to blame yourself for the collateral damage.
You are allowed to forgive yourself. Guilt and self-hate will do no one any good, the least of all you.
No one is right all the time. And no one has to hate themselves for mistakes they now have no power to change.
Breathe, move on, and let the past be where it is. It is no longer in your hands, but your present is. Don't fuck it up over that one mistake you committed when you didn't know any better.

9. Spending On Things or Experiences We Enjoy Doesn't Mean We Are Incapable of Saving Money
Growing up, my family was not very rich. Eating out and going on vacations were rare treats, and the children were always encouraged to save as much money as they can. As a result, we used our pencils and erasers to the last millimetre, wore our clothes till they were torn

or worn out, and never asked for anything that wasn't absolutely necessary.

This belief remained ingrained in me even as an adult. I went through college living on the bare minimum and not regretting it. But when I started working, there was this one time when a group of colleagues planned a weekend getaway to a nearby hill-station.

My knee-jerk reaction was to say, "No" without even knowing WHY I had refused.

I could easily afford the money and the time for the trip, but even then, why did I not go along with the plan?

In a moment, the truth hit me — it all came down to my conditioning. I was so used to saving up every penny I could, that allowing myself small pleasures felt like I was being irresponsible.

Un-learning this lesson was the most difficult, but, with time and repeated practice, I managed to outgrow it.

If you are in the same boat as me, then let me tell you that you don't have to feel guilty about spending on things and experiences that make you happy.

Yes, you are allowed to splurge on that stunning wedding dress you had your eyes on for months. You are entitled to go on that 14-day trip to Tuscany with your partner. Spending money on small indulgences is not wrong, as long as you spend responsibly.

Maintain a savings account. Learn about personal finance (or hire an expert). Keep an amount separate for emergencies. And you are free to spend the rest of the money in whichever pursuit of pleasure you want.

10. Having Fun Doesn't Mean We Are Irresponsible

We can take breaks. You can allot time and energy in doing things that satisfy your soul. Just because your parents worked so hard that they barely had time to relax, doesn't mean you deserve the same.

Burning yourself out and working till you drop down dead is not the only route to financial success.

Take out time for yourself. Breathe. Indulge in a hobby, anything that makes your chest feel light.

But when you do this, don't go overboard.

Plan out your day beforehand so that even after all your tasks are complete, you have time left to spend on self-care.

Maintain a journal and list your priorities for the day. Make sure you include time for yourself there.

Prioritise self-care. Buy that set of scented candles that you worry might make you look silly in front of the store cashier. Get a professional massage session. Lie down, put on that face pack, close your eyes, and relax.

You are allowed to take breaks. And no, it does not mean you are lying to yourself or not reaching your full potential.

You're being you. And sometimes, that's all you need to do.

Image for post

Photo by Giulia Bertelli on Unsplash

11. Wanting Sex Is Not Shameful

India is a country of 1.3 billion people and 0 sex education. All my life, the only lesson my mother gave me was that sex is evil, and I should refrain from it till I am married. That my virginity is precious and I should safeguard it and gift it only to my husband and no one else. If I fail to do so, no man would ever want me, and I would have to die alone.

I was young. Without realising, I had internalised this belief.

Fast forward to when I had my first boyfriend in college, and he wanted to get intimate. My mind said no, but my body wanted it. I had to exercise a herculean level of self-control and turn him down.

But, even then, later at night alone in my bed, I was racked with feelings of shame and guilt. I had been on the verge of giving it all to him. How could I be so irresponsible to want something so evil? How I could I betray my parents and my future husband this way?

It took years of re-wiring my mentality to reconcile my thoughts with what my body wanted. And if you have been trained to think along the same lines as I was, this is for you: no matter what the world might have led you to believe, the desires of your body are not evil. Carnal desires are just a way of celebrating the madness and mess that you are as a person. Holding back is like telling the universe you don't want to experience the gifts it has so generously bestowed on you.

12. Intimacy Doesn't Have to Lead to Heartbreak

All of us might have had bad experiences in the past where we gave all our love, time, and effort to one person, only to have them deny it, leaving us in a pool of our own self-pity and wasted dreams.

Relationships fail, and most often, there is nothing you can do to save them.

What you can do is not let a failed relationship define love for you.

John was a liar and a cheater. That does not mean all men are liars and cheaters. Sally had another man all this while, and you never knew. That does not mean all women have back-up options ready and will run off whenever you no longer offer them a "fair deal".

If you want to experience soul-stirring love, you have to keep your heart open to finding it, embracing it. Building walls around yourself to protect your heart will only lead you to miss out all the wonderful people in the world who might be there right at the next corner.

The world is full of awesome, loving people, and you are capable of attracting them to you. Don't close your heart because of one failed relationship. You are in control of your love life, and when you choose to love and be loved. Nothing and nobody can stop you.

13. Admitting That We're Sad, Tired, or Sick Doesn't Mean We're Weak

Another pitfall of growing up in a middle-class Indian family is watching your parents get tired, but, keep a strong face "for the sake of the family". My father would go to work each day, no matter how exhausted he felt. My mother cooked three meals for a family of four every single day without fail, even on days she was feeling under the weather. Seeing my parents work so hard imprinted this lesson deep in my brain: work is of the utmost importance. Anyone who shies away from work is weak.

But in truth, it is not.

You are allowed to skip work when you are sick. You are permitted to cancel plans when you are tired. You are entitled to seek help when you are unwell.

Knowing your strengths is excellent. But accepting your weaknesses, embracing them, and adjusting your life around them is even more liberating.

The ideas presented here are distilled from many centuries of efforts by many brilliant people. They are known all over the world, in diffuse, scattered form. Just knowing, understanding, and agreeing with, the concepts will not change much below the surface of the mind-heart.The use of this method will not do what you want to get done. It will make you better.

Chapter-3
The Power of Prayer

The prayer to be a positive mental exercise, something that lets you talk out your fears, feel better about a bad situation, etc. Those are true as well!

However, the power of prayer goes even deeper than that. I was raised in a religious family as a member of the Church of Jesus Christ of Latter-Day Saints. When I was in middle school, I started to seriously reflect, ponder and work out if in reality what I had been taught as a child was really true and something I wanted to dedicate my life too. More specifically I wanted to know if someone was actually listening to me pray day and night, does God really exist and would he answer me? Needless to say, I decided to get on my knees and pray, with real intent, or in other words, ready to follow whatever answer I received.

I stand as a witness that God answered my prayer. Not a vision or a voice of any sort but an unmistakable answer that I was being listened too, that he loved me and that I knew what I had been taught as a child was true.

That experience along with countless others have demonstrated to me that there is real and tangible power in reaching out to the Supreme Being that always is reaching out to you. Never hesitate to pray! Because there is a God I know that Satan is real and he does not want us to be happy or have the support of a loving God.

If nothing else, follow James's council in the New Testament, James 1:5. You lose nothing by connecting to the Lord but stand to gain everything.

However I no longer doubt prayer's effectiveness. I just doubt I was praying for the right things. Once I had my life-changing experience and found God and knew him for myself, I became utterly convinced of his existence as well as convinced of some things about religion. One is prayer. The primary purpose of prayer is to put us in communion with our soul, with the universe, with God, with all of those as a whole. In this state, we can communicate easily with ourselves and we can ask for what we really need and be sure of getting it. If we ask. And if we ask for what we really need and not what we think we want. And tell ourselves the truths we need to hear. "I am loved. I deserve to be loved. I will do good things for myself. I will help myself." Affirmations and guided meditation is another form of prayer. Trying talk to your deepest self and change what it believes. To be truly effective though, we need to know exactly what we're afraid of and exactly what we need to hear to motivate us.

I have evidence of the power of self-talk. I am getting happier as a result of remembering to tell myself good things and doing good things for myself.

One way to think about it is that God is the light. He shines love down on all of us to help us live and thrive.

In the most general sense, prayer is an act of worship that seeks to activate a rapport with the divine through deliberate communication, and this may or may not include an invocation in the process. Either way, the act of praying has been an essential part of what it means to be human for quite a while. There is a longstanding mystical tradition of praying which dates back tens of thousands of years. As part of this ancient legacy of devotion, I have prayed with my father and he with his, and so on and so forth, all the way back to the first recognition of divinity nearly four thousand generations ago.

Granted, depending on how and why people pray, the act itself might either be individual or communal and could take place in public or in private. There really is no limit to the different kinds of spirituality and religiosity that can emerge. In regards to this, spirituality is for the soul while religiosity is for God. To better understand what I mean by this it's important to realize that a long time ago all of the indigenous people on the habitable continents were animists. This formed the basis of their spirituality. So, from their point of view communication with both embodied and disembodied souls was essential to their way of life. As a result of this, in line with the customs of their local tribe, a shaman would enter trance states in an effort to gain better access to metaphysical space. Then, religiosity eventually grew out of that spirituality. This inevitably gave rise to countless different creation myths among early humans.

Dozens of millennia later, monotheism has become the dominant form of both spirituality and religiosity in the world. However, the act of praying has evolved and it will continue to do so as the soul improves over time. God only knows what we might do next. For now, observant Jews currently pray three times a day, with lengthier sessions on certain occasions, such as the Shabbat and during the reading of the Torah. Then again, in yet another example of the Abrahamic faiths, the command to ritual prayer is mentioned in several of the Surahs in the Qur'an. Prayer is absolutely vital to Muslims. In the religion of Islam there are five daily obligatory prayers that are required for Salat which is one of the five pillars of their faith.

Meanwhile, Hindus have a very different form of worship. Regardless, as part of their religion, once a year in India tens of millions of devotees of several Eastern traditions come together in the largest congregation on the planet. There, at the confluence of three sacred rivers where Sadhus sit smoking Ganja, people of all ages celebrate their faith together as one. This incredibly holy festival currently consists of the biggest prayer group on Earth. Although in all likelihood the Muslims will hold the record in the not-too-distant future. As another of the five pillars of their faith, the Hajj is an annual pilgrimage to Mecca that has been drawing a bigger crowd with each passing year and the trend shows no signs of slowing down anytime soon. Enormous congregations like this are magnificent achievements for humanity, either way. More importantly, they offer us glimpses of the kind of overwhelmingly glorious global piety that our species could one day achieve.

Now, don't get me wrong, it's really important for everyone to understand that this isn't just about doing something at certain times, or in special places, in tremendously spectacular ways. That's not really the point at all, although those things are still very important. Instead, occasions such as those should serve as reminders for us to always live with a positive spiritual and religious attitude. With that in mind, the act of saying grace before meals is something everyone might want to do just as an easy way to incorporate God into what they already do on a daily basis. No matter what, the point is that it's very important for everyone to make room for the Supreme Being in their lives. Ultimately, prayer is simply about making yourself available to God, while at the same time making God available to you.

The power of prayer should not be underestimated. "The prayer of a righteous man is powerful and effective. Elijah was a man just like us. He prayed earnestly that it would not rain, and it did not rain on the land for three and a half years. Again he prayed, and the heavens gave rain, and the earth produced its crops." God most definitely listens to prayers, answers prayers, and moves in response to prayers.

Jesus taught, "…I tell you the truth, if you have faith as small as a mustard seed, you can say to this mountain, 'Move from here to there' and it will move. Nothing will be impossible for you"
"The weapons we fight with are not the weapons of the world. On the contrary, they have divine power to demolish strongholds. We demolish arguments and every pretension that sets itself up against the knowledge of God, and we take captive every thought to make it obedient to Christ." The Bible urges us, "And pray in the Spirit on all occasions with all kinds of prayers and requests. With this in mind, be alert and always keep on praying for all the saints"

Power Of Prayer - How do I tap into it?
The power of prayer is not the result of the person praying. Rather, the power resides in the God who is being prayed to.

"This is the confidence we have in approaching God: that if we ask anything according to his will, he hears us. And if we know that he hears us - whatever we ask - we know that we have what we asked of him." No matter the person praying, the passion behind the prayer, or the purpose of the prayer - God answers prayers that are in agreement with His will. His answers are not always yes, but are always in our best interest. When our desires line up with His will, we will come to understand that in time. When we pray passionately and purposefully, according to God's will, God responds powerfully!

We cannot access powerful prayer by using "magic formulas." Our prayers being answered is not based on the eloquence of our prayers. We don't have to use certain words or phrases to get God to answer our prayers. In fact, Jesus rebukes those who pray using repetitions, "And when you pray, do not keep on babbling like pagans, for they think they will be heard because of their many words. Do not be like them, for your Father knows what you need before you ask him" Prayer is communicating with God. All you have to do is ask God for His help.
 "Then they cried out to the LORD in their trouble, and he brought them out of their distress. He stilled the storm to a whisper; the waves of the sea were hushed. They were glad when it grew calm, and he guided them to their desired haven." There is power in prayer!

Power Of Prayer - For what kind of things should I pray?

God's help through the power of prayer is available for all kinds of requests and issues. "Do not be anxious about anything, but in everything, by prayer and petition, with thanksgiving, present your requests to God. And the peace of God, which transcends all understanding, will guard your hearts and your minds in Christ Jesus."

 The Lord's prayer is not a prayer we are supposed to memorize and simply recite to God. It is only an example of how to pray and the things that should go into a prayer - worship, trust in God, requests, confession, protection, etc. Pray for these kinds of things, but speak to God using your own words.

The Word of God is full of accounts describing the power of prayer in various situations. The power of prayer has overcome enemies, conquered death. God, through prayer, opens eyes, changes hearts, heals wounds, and grants wisdom The power of prayer should never be underestimated because it draws on the glory and might of the infinitely powerful God of the universe!

"All the peoples of the earth are regarded as nothing. He does as he pleases with the powers of heaven and the peoples of the earth. No one can hold back his hand or say to him: 'What have you done?'"

Chapter-4
The Power of Gratitude

Benefits of Gratitude:

There are numerous benefits of practicing Gratitude.

We will build a powerful daily gratitude habit and re-discover all the great things that are already in our life.

1. Gratitude makes us happier.

A five-minute a daily gratitude journal can increase your long-term well-being by more than 10 percent.

That's the same impact as doubling your income!

How can a free five-minute activity compare? Gratitude improves our health, relationships, emotions, personality, and career.

Sure, having more money can be pretty awesome, but because of hedonic adaptation we quickly get used to it and stop having as much fun and happiness as we did at first.

Gratitude makes us feel more gratitude.

This is why a five-minute a week gratitude journal can make us so much happier. The actual gratitude produced during those five minutes is small, but the emotions of gratitude felt during those five-minutes are enough to trigger a grateful mood.

While in a grateful mood, we will feel gratitude more frequently, when we do feel gratitude it will be more intense and held for longer, and we will feel gratitude for more things at the same time.

In five words – gratitude triggers positive feedback loops.

Hedonic what?

After repeated exposure to the same emotion-producing stimulus, we tend to experience less of the emotion. Put more simply, we get use to the good things that happen to us. This also means that we get used to the bad things that happen to us. Those who have been disabled have a remarkable ability to rebound – initially, they may feel terrible, but after months or years, they are on average just as happy as everyone else.

Hedonic adaptation gives unparalleled resiliency and keeps us motivated to achieve even greater things. It also kills our marriages – we get used to our amazing spouse (or kids, or job, or house, or car, or game). We stop seeing as much positive and start complaining. It is a psychological imperative to fight hedonic adaptation if we want to maximize happiness. Gratitude is one of the most powerful tools in our arsenal.

Why does it take several months?

In all relevant studies, changes occurred slowly. It took several months of continuous practice for the largest benefits to appear. This is for two reasons:

Cultivating gratitude is a skill. After three months of practice, I now have the ability to self-generate slight feelings of gratitude and happiness on command. With more time and practice, I expect the intensity and duration of the generated feelings to increase. Gratitude is a personality trait. Some people have more grateful personalities than others. Daily gratitude practice can change our personality, but that takes a long time.

2. Gratitude makes people like us.

Gratitude generates social capital – in two studies with 243 total participants, those who were 10% more grateful than average had 17.5% more social capital.

Gratitude makes us nicer, more trusting, more social, and more appreciative. As a result, it helps us make more friends, deepen our existing relationships, and improve our marriage.

3. Gratitude makes us healthier.

There is even reason to believe gratitude can extend your lifespan by a few months or even years.

4. Gratitude boosts our career.

Gratitude makes you a more effective manager,

helps you network, increases your decision-making capabilities, increases your productivity, and helps you get mentors and proteges.

As a result, gratitude helps you achieve your career goals, as well as making your workplace a more friendly and enjoyable place to be.

Do you think this is effective?

I'm not suggesting that criticism and self-focus don't have a place in the workplacc, but I think we're overdoing it.

5. Gratitude strengthens our emotions.

Gratitude reduces feelings of envy, makes our memories happier, lets us experience good feelings, and helps us bounce back from stress.

6. Gratitude develops our personality.

It really does, and in potentially life-changing ways.

If you're a man, don't worry; gratitude won't transform you into a woman

7. Gratitude makes us more optimistic.

Gratitude is strongly correlated with optimism. Optimism in turn makes us happier, improves our health, and has been shown to increase lifespan by as much as a few years.

I'd say a 5 minute a day gratitude journal would be worth it just for this benefit.

In one study of keeping a weekly gratitude journal, participants showed a 5% increase in optimism. In another study, keeping a daily gratitude journal resulted in a 15% increase in optimism. Optimism is significantly correlated with gratitude.

How does gratitude increase optimism?

The act of gratitude is the act of focusing on the good in life. If we perceive our current life to have more good, we will also believe our future life to have more good. Optimism is correlated with gratitude because those with an optimistic disposition are biologically more likely to focus on the good (gratitude) than on the bad (personal disappointment, anxiety, etc…).

8. Gratitude reduces materialism.

Why is materialism negatively correlated with happiness and well-being?

Materialism is strongly correlated with reduced well-being and increased rates of mental disorder.

There's nothing wrong with wanting more. The problem with materialism is that it makes people feel less competent, reduces feelings of relatedness and gratitude, reduces their ability to appreciate and enjoy the good in life, generates negative emotions, and makes them more self-centered.

The pursuit of wealth and power has been shown in dozens of studies to be a highly inefficient method of increasing well-being and happiness. To be sure, if your income doubles you will be slightly happier. But how much effort do you think is involved in doubling your income? How many sacrifices are required? Motivational speakers will tell you that the money is worth the sacrifices. I disagree.

Applying that same level of energy towards strengthening one's relationships, cultivating compassion and gratitude, and so on much more reliably creates positive, transformative change.

Said differently, material success is not a very important factor in the happiness of highly grateful people.

How does gratitude reduce materialism?

Materialism flows from two sources: role models and insecurity.

Americans are inundated with materialistic role models every day: from advertisements which highlight materialistic themes, to celebrity culture which glorifies the rich and frivolous, to business culture in which we are told our dreams should be to be rich and powerful. Gratitude helps by reducing our tendency to compare ourselves to those with a higher social status. Those who are insecure, that is, those that have not had their basic psychological needs met (e.g. those who lack confidence, come from a poor background, or had unsupportive parents), are more likely to be materialistic. Gratitude is an effective strategy for reducing insecurity. A grateful emotion is triggered when we perceive an act of benevolence directed towards us. Those who are dispositionally ungrateful are therefore less likely to perceive acts of benevolence, even if they are surrounded by a loving environment. Flipped around, those who cultivate an attitude of gratitude are more likely to perceive an environment of benevolence, which in turn causes their brains to assume they are in an environment full of

social support, which in turn kills insecurity and materialism.
Will gratitude make me lazy?

Those who are more materialistic are more likely to relentlessly pursue wealth. So while gratitude won't make you lazy, over your lifetime you may end up earning less money. You will instead re-focus on other things. You may, for example, spend time with friends, family, and your hobbies. That's a good thing.

Regret #2: Working too hard.

Gratitude has caused me to focus less on things that don't matter, like making money, and more on the things that do, like my family and this blog. I think that's a good thing.

9. Gratitude increases spiritualism.

Spiritual transcendence is highly correlated with feelings of gratitude. That is – the more spiritual you are, the more likely you are to be grateful.

This is for two reasons:

All major religions espouse gratitude as a virtue. Spirituality spontaneously gives rise to grateful behavior. I believe the opposite to also be true, that gratitude spontaneously gives rise to spiritual attribution, helping one feel closer to God or other religious entities. I am irreligious, and have found gratitude practices to make my spiritual position difficult – those moments when I feel intense gratitude make me want to believe in a benevolent God. My solution has been to re-direct my feelings towards Lady Luck.

Why does spirituality give rise to grateful behavior?

Many of the sub-traits associated with spirituality are the same sub-traits associated with gratitude. For example, spiritual individuals are more likely to feel a strong spiritual or emotional connection with others, and to believe in inter-connectedness. Both are prerequisites for feeling gratitude – someone who feels weak connections with others, and who believes in the illusion of self-sufficiency is unlikely to feel gratitude.

10. Gratitude makes us less self-centered.

I'll be totally honest, I'm a self-centered twat. I'm a lot better now that I've brought gratitude into my life, but I still spend way too much time thinking about myself, and too little thinking about others. I expect this to change – because of my compassion and gratitude practices I am starting to have spontaneous urges to help others.

This is because the very nature of gratitude is to focus on others (on their acts of benevolence). In this regard, gratitude practice can be better than self-esteem therapy. Self-esteem therapy focuses the individual back on themselves: I'm smart, I look good, I can succeed, etc.…

That can work, but it can also make us narcissistic or even back-fire and lower self-esteem.

11. Gratitude increases self-esteem.

Imagine a world where no one helps you. Despite your asking and pleading, no one helps you.

Now imagine a world where many people help you all of the time for no other reason than that they like you. In which world do you think you would have more self-esteem? Gratitude helps to create a world like that.

How does gratitude create a more supportive social dynamic?

Gratitude does this in two ways:

Gratitude has been shown in multiple studies to make people kinder and more friendly, and that because of that, grateful people have more social capital. This means that grateful people are actually more likely to receive help from others for no reason other than that they are liked and appreciated.
Gratitude increases your recognition of benevolence. For example, a person with low self-esteem may view an act of kindness with a skeptical eye, thinking that the benefactor is trying to get something from them. A

grateful person would take the kindness at face value, believing themselves to be a person worthy of receiving no-strings-attached kindness.
Health

12. Gratitude improves our sleep.

Gratitude increases sleep quality, reduces the time required to fall asleep, and increases sleep duration. Said differently, gratitude can help with insomnia.

The key is what's on our minds as we're trying to fall asleep. If it's worries about the kids, or anxiety about work, the level of stress in our body will increase, reducing sleep quality, keeping us awake, and cutting our sleep short.

If it's thinking about a few things we have to be grateful for today, it will induce the relaxation response, knock us out, and keep us that way.

Yes – gratitude is a (safe and free) sleep aid.

I don't believe you!

In one study of 65 subjects with a chronic pain condition, those who were assigned a daily gratitude journal to be completed at night reported half an hour more sleep than the control group.

In another study of 400 healthy people, those participants who had higher scores on a gratitude test also had significantly better sleep. They reported faster time to sleep, improved sleep quality, increased sleep duration, and less difficulty staying awake during the day.

This is not because their life was simply better – levels of gratitude are more dependent on personality and life perspective than on life situation.

13. Gratitude keeps us away from the doctor.

Gratitude can't cure cancer (neither can positive-thinking), but it can strengthen your physiological functioning.

Positive emotion improves health. The details are complicated, but the overall picture is not – if you want to improve your health, improve your mind.

Gratitude is a positive emotion. It's no far stretch that some of the benefits (e.g. better coping & management of terminal conditions like cancer and HIV,

faster recovery from certain medical procedures, positive changes in immune system functioning,

more positive health behavior,

etc…) apply to gratitude as well.

In fact, some recent science shows just that – those who engage in gratitude practices have been shown to feel less pain, go to the doctor less often, have lower blood pressure, and be less likely to develop a mental disorder.

How does gratitude improve my health?

The science on how is still unclear. Here are two ideas:

Gratitude reduces levels of stress by activating the parasympathetic nervous system. Stress in turn has been shown to disrupt healthy body functioning (e.g disrupting the hypothalamic-pituitary axis, the immune system, our sleep, etc…).
Gratitude encourages pro-health behavior like exercising and paying attention to health risks.
14. Gratitude lets us live longer.

I will be honest with you – by combining the results of a few different studies I'm confident that gratitude can extend lifespan, but no single study as yet has actually proven this claim.

Here is what we know: optimism and positive emotion, in general, have been used to successfully predict mortality decades later.

The optimistic lived a few years longer than the pessimistic. A few years may not sound like much, but I know when I'm about to die I'd like to have a few more years!

We also know that gratitude is strongly correlated with positive emotion. So, gratitude –> positive emotion –> an extra few months or years on earth. With positive psychology research on the rise, I believe we can expect this claim to be rigorously tested within the next five to ten years.

15. Gratitude increases our energy levels.

Gratitude and vitality are strongly correlated – the grateful are much more likely to report physical and mental vigor.

Study of 238 people found a correlation between vitality and gratitude.This means that vitality and gratitude are strongly correlated even after considering the possibility that they are correlated because high-energy people and high-gratitude people share personality traits like extroversion in common.
Do people with more energy tend to experience more gratitude, does gratitude lead to increased energy, or is something else going on?

I believe it's two of those three:

People with high levels of vitality tend to have some of the same traits that highly grateful people do, like high levels of optimism and life satisfaction.

Gratitude increases physical and mental well-being, which in turn increases energy levels.

16. Gratitude makes us more likely to exercise.

In one 11-week study of 96 Americans, those who were instructed to keep a weekly gratitude journal exercised 40 minutes more per week.

Once again, time will tell – but it would not surprise me if being grateful for one's health would increase one's tendency to want to protect it by exercising more.

17. Gratitude helps us bounce back.

Those that have more gratitude have a more pro-active coping style, are more likely to have and seek out social support in times of need, are less likely to develop PTSD, and are more likely to grow in times of stress.

In others words, they are more resilient.

18. Gratitude makes us feel good.

Surprise, surprise: gratitude actually feels good. Yet only 20% of Americans rate gratitude as a positive and constructive emotion (compared to 50% of Europeans).

According to gratitude researcher Kabir Emmons, gratitude is just happiness that we recognize after-the fact to have been caused by the kindness of others. Gratitude doesn't just make us happier, it is happiness in and of itself!

That's no surprise – we idealize the illusion of self-sufficiency. Gratitude, pah! That's for the weak.

Gratitude feels good, and if the benefits on this page are any indication – gratitude will make us stronger, healthier, and more successful.

Are we afraid to admit that luck, God, family members, friends, and/or strangers have and will continue to strongly influence your life? I once was – not only was I less happy, I was also weaker. It takes strength to admit to the truth of inter-dependency.

19. Gratitude makes our memories happier.

Our memories are not set in stone, like data stored on a hard-drive. There are dozens of ways our memories get changed over time – we remember things as being worse than they actually were, as being longer or shorter, people as being kinder or crueler, as being more or less interesting, and so on.

Experiencing gratitude in the present makes us more likely to remember positive memories,

and actually transforms some of our neutral or even negative memories into positive ones.

In one study, putting people into a grateful mood helped them find closure of upsetting open memories.

During these experiences, participants were more likely to recall positive aspects of the memory than usual, and some of the negative and neutral aspects were transformed into positives.

What's going on with my memory!?

It's called cognitive biases. Here are two great books on the subject: Thinking, Fast and Slow (written by the founder of behavioral economics, Daniel Kahneman), and Mistakes Were Made (But Not by Me).

20. Gratitude reduces feelings of envy.

A small bit of jealousy or envy directed at the right target is motivating. Too much produces feelings of insecurity, materialism, inferiority, distrust, and unhappiness.

How does gratitude reduce feelings of envy?

The personality trait of envy has a correlation of -.39 with the personality trait of gratitude. In addition, on days when people experience more gratitude, they are also more likely to experience less envy.

This is likely because an attitude of envy and an attitude of gratitude are largely incompatible. Just like it is impossible to feel optimistic and pessimistic at the same time, gratitude is the act of perceiving benevolence, while envy and jealousy is the act of perceiving inadequacy. Benevolence and inadequacy cannot be completely perceived at the same time.

21. Gratitude helps us relax.

Gratitude and positive emotion in general are among the strongest relaxants known to man. I was having trouble sleeping a few nights ago because I was too stressed and couldn't relax. I'll be honest, for the few minutes that I was able to hold feelings of gratitude I almost fell asleep, but holding feelings of gratitude is hard! In this case, too hard – I ended up getting out of bed.

Gratitude may be just as or even more effective than relaxation methods such as deep breathing, but because it is also more difficult, is unfeasible as an actual relaxation technique. Think of it like tea – one or two cups help you relax – three of four make you want to empty your bladder. But it could just be me. Perhaps you'll find practices of gratitude more natural and easy.

Social

22. Gratitude makes us friendlier.

Multiple studies have shown that gratitude induces pro-social behavior. Keeping a gratitude journal is enough to make you more likely to help others with their problems and makes you more likely to offer them emotional support.

Why?

There are two main reasons.

Gratitude helps us perceive kindness, which we have a natural tendency to want to reciprocate. Without the feeling of gratitude, we may not recognize when someone is helping us (the same way anger lets us know when someone is trying to harm us).
Gratitude makes us happier and more energetic, both of which are highly linked to pro-social behavior.
23. Gratitude helps your marriage.

I've never been married, but from what I've heard, read, and seen, one-way marriages start to suffer is that when the passion starts to fizzle, the partners become less appreciative and naggier.

Scientists have put numbers to our intuition and experience, creating an appreciation to naggy ratio. More formally called the Losada ratio, it divides the total number of positive expressions (support, encouragement and appreciation) made during a typical interaction by the number of negative expressions (disapproval, sarcasm, and cynicism).

When the ratio was below .9, that is there were 11% more negative expressions than positive expressions, marriages plummeted towards divorce or languishment. Those marriages that lasted and were found satisfying were those with a positivity ratio above 5.1 (five positive expressions to each negative).

Building regular practices of gratitude into your marriage is an easy but effective way of raising your positivity ratio.

Correlation or causality?

Does the positivity ratio actually change the dynamics of a marriage, or does it simply reflect underlying happiness or conflict? Would 'faking' a higher positivity ratio actually change the dynamics of your marriage, or would it be the same as faking your income on a survey – it may let you temporarily feel better, but it doesn't actually make you any richer?

There is a reason to believe it is both. What we say and how we act becomes who we are. Faking a smile has been shown to actually make people happier. But the effect is only so strong. I believe that for gratitude to truly affect a marriage, it must come from the heart. With enough practice and effort, it can.

P.S. You shouldn't take the numbers too literally. A good rule of thumb is three or four positives for each negative means you're doing well.

24. Gratitude makes us look good.

Ingratitude is universally regarded with contempt. It's opposite, gratitude is considered a virtue in all major religions and most modern cultures. It may not be sexy to be grateful, but people will respect you for it.

Gratitude is not the same thing as indebtedness, which we rightly avoid. Indebtedness is a negative emotion which carries an assumption of repayment.

Gratitude is not the same thing as weakness. Weakness is flattery or subservience.

Gratitude is the acknowledgment of kindness with thanks.

It takes big balls to acknowledge that we didn't get to where we are all on our own – that without others we may never have made it. That's why, just maybe, gratitude may be sexy too.

25. Gratitude helps us make friends.

When I was in college I found it really easy to make new friends. If I hadn't moved out of NYC it would still be easy – living in a farm town makes it difficult. I've found an effective way to start a conversation or move a relationship forward is an expression of gratitude, "thank you for that coffee, it was super delicious." *wink, wink*

Ah, my mistake – that's actually what I use to hit on my barista.

But you get the point.

26. Gratitude deepens friendships.

I have one friend who always deeply thanks me for taking the time to see her. That makes me feel appreciated and that makes me feel good. Wouldn't it make you feel good too?

Career

27. Gratitude makes us a more effective manager.

Effective management requires a toolbox of skills. Criticism comes all too easily to most, while the ability to feel gratitude and express praise is often lacking.

Timely, sincere, specific, behavior-focused praise is often a more powerful method of influencing change than criticism. Specifically, multiple studies have found expressions of gratitude to be highly motivating, while expressions of criticism to be slightly de-motivating but providing more expectation clarification.

Contrary to expectation, if praise is moderate and behavior focused, repeat expressions of gratitude will not lose their impact, and employee performance will increase.

Because of our culture, expressions of gratitude are often difficult to give – cultivating an attitude of gratitude will help.

I've seen firsthand the powerful difference between interacting with subordinates more with praise, and interacting with some more with criticism. Those I've given more praise are more enthusiastic about working with me, express more creativity, and are so much more fun to work with.

28. Gratitude helps us build our network.

Gratitude has been shown across a number of studies to increase social behavior. Two longitudinal studies showed that those with higher levels of gratitude actually developed more social capital than those with lower levels.

Gratitude helps you get mentors, proteges, and benefactors.

Those who are more grateful are more likely to help others, and to pay it forward, that is, to take on mentoring relationships. But I'm guessing you care more about getting help from mentors and benefactors than being a mentor yourself. Well, that makes sense – having one or more mentors dramatically increases one's success rate.

The first level is simple – those who are grateful are more social and also more likely to ask for help. But it goes one step further – we all ask for help at one time, one of the key differences between one-off help and establishing a mentoring relationship is gratitude.

Flipped around, what is it that makes a person want to help you on a continuous basis? Gratitude – when their wisdom, experience, and time are well appreciated, mentors will find enjoyment from the process, continuing to help you for weeks, months, or years.

29. Gratitude increases our goal achievement.

In one study, participants were asked to write down those goals which they wished to accomplish over the next two months. Those who were instructed to keep a gratitude journal reported more progress on achieving their goals at the end of the study. One result doesn't make science – what you should take away from this is that, at the least, gratitude will not make you lazy and passive. It might even do the opposite!

30. Gratitude improves our decision making.

Decision making is really tiring – so tiring that we automate to our subconscious much of the reasoning that goes behind making a decision. Even for the most basic of decisions, like where to go eat, there are dozens of variables to consider: how much time and money do I want to spend, what cuisine would I like today, am I willing to travel far, what should I get once I get there, and so on. If you deliberated on each of these decisions one at a time, your mind would be overwhelmed.

The problem gets even worse for more complex decisions like making a diagnosis.

In one study, doctors were given a list of ailments from a hypothetical patient and also given a misleading piece of information—that the patient had been diagnosed at another hospital as having lupus. Half the doctors had gratitude evoked by giving them a token of appreciation. Those who did not receive a token of appreciation were more likely to stick with the incorrect diagnosis of lupus; those who did receive the gratitude were energized to expend more energy and to pay their gratitude forward onto their patient. They also considered a wider range of treatment options.

 shows that gratitude motivates improved decision making. Those who cultivate an attitude of gratitude find tokens of appreciation every day, on their own.

31. Gratitude increases our productivity.

Those who are insecure have difficulty focusing because many of their mental resources are tied up with their worries. On the other hand, those who are highly confident are able to be more productive, because they can direct more of their focus towards their work. This operates at both a conscious and subconscious level – we may be getting mentally distracted by our worries, or more commonly, parts of our subconscious mind are expending energy to suppress negative information and concerns.

As gratitude has been shown to increase self-esteem and reduce insecurity, this means that it can help us focus and improve our productivity.

Chapter-5
Law of Attraction to deal with Stress

The law of attraction is very powerful. With belief anything can be achieved. Without it, nothing is possible.

"Whether a man thinks he can or he can't, he's right" - Henry Ford

So right from the start you can determine where someone will go and what they can achieve. Over time with belief you can create amazing things. With the same time and carrying disbelief, you can 'cut' yourself off from many achievements.

Most people create through default. Their thoughts aren't always aligned with their deepest desires. They don't believe they are possible. Or, they create a middle ground which is more in line with their conflicting beliefs or their laziness!

Either way, the law of attraction is working; bringing the fruits of your perpetual thinking processes to life. When my son, Kabir, was in the second grade, we lived in a small town in northern California among the giant redwood trees. It is a community known for its peacefulness and unity, the land of vegans and tree-huggers. People there value togetherness and acceptance.

At this time, I was studying "The Secret" by Rhonda Byrne, a movie and book that introduced many to the Law of Attraction. I would watch the movie daily, taking notes and comparing different aspects of the lessons involved. This was a bit different than my family was used to as most of my previous study involved just books and reading, which Kabir was not interested in. He often sat with me and watched the movie, though.

After watching the movie several times, Kabir started asking questions. He wanted to know, as boys do, what dad was up to. We talked at great length about the law and how it shaped our lives.

One day he came home from school and announced that his class would be studying fossils. Kabir asked me if we could go buy a fossil so he could have his own. I explained to him that I did not know of a place that sold fossils, but we could look into it. He thought for a moment and said, "Why don't we just use the Law of Attraction to get one"?

I froze. My thoughts and feelings of disbelief took over, and I started to think of a way to talk him out of this idea. Before I could speak, he announced that he did not need my help. He was going to get a fossil the "Secret" way, on his own.

We quickly reviewed the basic principles, and he was off. I really thought it would end there. I was wrong.

A few days later, Kabir was playing in the yard, and he wanted to play in the rock garden. He asked for my help to move some particularly heavy stones, and while we re-arranged the rocks, he commented that the one he was holding was actually a fossilized piece of wood. I commented on the fact that he had requested of the universe a fossil, and here it was!

He was having none of that. "No, dad, this is not mine. This is not the fossil I requested. I will know it when I see it."

The next day, when I picked him up from school, his teacher (we'll call her Mrs. G) asked me to stay for a minute to discuss something. She gingerly reported that Kabir had told the class that he was going to get a real fossil of his own using the Law of Attraction. She was a great teacher and cared for her students as if they were her own. The best. And she was worried that he would be disappointed when this fossil did not arrive.

I smiled at her and asked how she thought he would feel if it did arrive. Could she believe it was possible? Several of the other parents gave disapproving looks, and Mrs. G tried to be helpful without violating my wishes as a parent. It was awkward, but I knew then as I do now that she had his best interest at heart. I asked her to have faith and see what happens.

Kabir continued his affirmations and visualizations, boldly claiming his prize was on the way. He KNEW it was coming.

About 2 weeks later, his teacher asked me to stay late again. She was bubbling! On Kabir's desk was a small package, and he was asked to open it. Inside were two small fossils. He shrieked when he opened the box and said, "Here they are, just as I asked! See, everyone!"

Mrs. G looked at me and quietly explained that she had written her professor in Washington state and had him send these to her for Kabir. With tears in her eyes, she thanked Kabir for restoring her faith. The other parents who had been so disapproving before took turns looking at the treasures in his hands. The look on his face said it all.

There are many things to be learned from this story. One of the most important for me is that the 'magic' that brings things about is not the kind a sorcerer produces, but rather the kind that LOVE produces. Was this magical? Absolutely. But the process is also very visible here. Kabir believed so strongly that he was able to 'attract' the needed people with the needed sympathetic vibration to make this happen. His belief radiated out and changed the thinking of others to bring about his desire.

Had he not believed so completely and openly, this would never have happened. This is where 'wishful thinking' and the Law of Attraction differ. Kabir's unquestioning belief caused action on his part, and in turn, action on the part of others.

To this day, Kabir treasures his fossils. Not because of what they are, but what they represent. He knows he can accomplish anything he puts his mind to, and that is a priceless gift to any human being. He is in high school now, but he still remembers this as being one of the happiest moments of his life.

The Law of Attraction uses many different ways to make things happen. An infinite number of ways, really. This is just one example, but it is a good one. He believed, and he took action - even if that action was merely to speak boldly about his intention. And he helped many others along the way without even meaning to.

It is not for us to determine the 'how', but to believe and act when actions are indicated. You never know how far-reaching your actions can go or how things will come about.

It's not magic, but it is magical.

The Law of Attraction—the concept that our thoughts and feelings create our experiences, and that we attract to ourselves what we focus our attention on—has a long history as a theory, but gained wide popularity due to "The Secret", Oprah, and other mass media outlets. While there are different theories of why it may work, and caveats you should be aware of, you can use the principles of the law of attraction to relieve stress and to attract the life you want. (I've used it in my practice and in my personal life, and it's worked for me.) The following steps can lead you to the less-stressed life you envision.

List Your Frustrations
Make a list of all the things in your life that have you feeling frustrated, or that you'd like to change. This can include a stressful job, your children's behavior, or conflict in your relationships, for example.

List the Positives
Next, begin a journal. For each situation on your list, find everything you can think of that's positive in the situation. For example, a difficult job may also bring the benefits of income, creative challenge, or personal growth; the job can be a vehicle for expanding your level of patience, for example. (At the very least, it could bring you the valuable information that this isn't what you want to be doing with your life!)

Maintain a Positive Attitude
This doesn't just mean to paste a smile on your face; it means to work at feeling grateful for what you already have, and for what you believe will come. That's right: shift your focus from your feelings of lack, and toward feelings of gratitude and abundance.

Believe in yourself, in your future, and in God or the universe, and know that you can make whatever changes in your life you want.

Visualize a Better Life
Building and maintaining a visual image of what you want in your life (instead of focusing on what you don't want) can be a powerful way to attract positive change and opportunity. Make a detailed list of what you'd like in your life. Sit down daily and visualize what your new life would look like and how it would feel to have these changes.

Think, Feel, Act
Be sure that your thoughts, feelings, and behavior all
focus on your goals, rather than your frustrations with
your situation, or any negative feelings you may have.
Keep your self-talk positive and optimistic; engage in
visualizations each day that reflect the life you want;
work on your plan of action. If you do this, you should
find you make quick strides in the life you want.

Tips: How to use it.
Frame your thoughts the way you would create positive
affirmations, by focusing on what you do want rather
than what frustrates you. (You can learn positive
affirmations for additional information on this effective
tool for positive change.)
Keep a gratitude journal, where you record the things
for which you are grateful. There are many health and
stress management benefits to journaling, and this
practice helps you develop an attitude of gratitude,
which creates a space for more abundance.
If you're not sure how your thoughts affect your life, you
can assess your thought patterns with an optimism
quiz.
Accept What Is. Rather than spending every day
focused on what you don't like about your life and
wishing things were different, try to come to terms with
the bad as well as the good. This doesn't mean that
you don't make positive changes in your life; it just
means you don't focus on your frustrations every day.
You make peace with what is while making progress
toward what you'd like to have.

Create Statements. Once you get an idea of what you're aiming for, try to put that idea into a few simple statements that reflect the reality of what you want to create. Phrase the statements as if they are already true, not that you would like them to be true. For example, the affirmation, "I am feeling more peaceful each day," would be better than, "I want to feel more peaceful." This is because you are programming your subconscious mind to believe the statements, and that helps manifest them into reality.

Some Affirmations to combat stress:
I'm cool, calm, confident and optimistic about my future.
I am everyday getting more confident, more enthusiastic and more powerful.

Once you've put together your collection of statements, here are some fun ways to introduce positive affirmations into your life.

Repetition. Probably the most popular way to harness the power of affirmations is to simply repeat them to yourself on a regular basis. Repeating them mentally several times in the morning or evening can be effective; repeating them aloud is even more effective because you hear them more clearly that way.

* 9 7 9 8 6 9 1 4 5 5 4 9 0 *